AF236380

Last Chance Viral Phage Therapy

The Natural Alternative to Antibiotics

Martin Scott

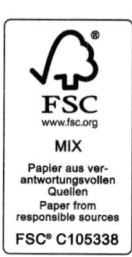

Bibliografische Information der Deutschen Nationalbibliothek:

Die Deutsche Nationalbibliothek verzeichnet diese Publikation in der Deutschen Nationalbibliografie; detaillierte bibliografische Daten sind im Internet über http://dnb.dnb.de abrufbar.

Herstellung und Verlag: BoD – Books on Demand, Norderstedt

ISBN: 978-3-7526-4103-5

Introduction

By using this book, you accept this disclaimer in full.

No advice

The book contains information. The information is not advice and should not be treated as such.

No representations or warranties

To the maximum extent permitted by applicable law and subject to section below, we exclude all representations, warranties, undertakings and guarantees relating to the book.

Without prejudice to the generality of the foregoing paragraph, we do not represent, warrant, undertake or guarantee:

- that the information in the book is correct, accurate, complete or non-misleading.

- that the use of the guidance in the book will lead to any particular outcome or result.

Limitations and exclusions of liability

The limitations and exclusions of liability set out in this section and elsewhere in this disclaimer: are subject to section 6 below; and govern all liabilities arising under the disclaimer or in relation to the book, including liabilities arising in contract, in tort (including negligence) and for breach of statutory duty.

We will not be liable to you in respect of any losses arising out of any event or events beyond our reasonable control.

We will not be liable to you in respect of any business losses, including without limitation loss of or damage to profits, income, revenue, use, production, anticipated savings, business, contracts, commercial opportunities or goodwill.

We will not be liable to you in respect of any loss or corruption of any data, database or software.

We will not be liable to you in respect of any special, indirect or consequential loss or damage.

Exceptions

Nothing in this disclaimer shall: limit or exclude our liability for death or personal injury resulting from negligence; limit or exclude our liability for fraud or fraudulent misrepresentation; limit any of our liabilities in any way that is not permitted under applicable law; or exclude any of our liabilities that may not be excluded under applicable law.

Severability

If a section of this disclaimer is determined by any court or other competent authority to be unlawful and/or unenforceable, the other sections of this disclaimer continue in effect.

If any unlawful and/or unenforceable section would be lawful or enforceable if part of it were deleted, that part will be deemed to be deleted, and the rest of the section will continue in effect.

Law and jurisdiction

This disclaimer will be governed by and construed in accordance with Swiss law, and any disputes relating to this disclaimer will be subject to the exclusive jurisdiction of the courts of Switzerland.

Contents

War against Antibiotic Resistant Bacteria 142

Conclusion 158

Introduction

The widespread nature of antibiotic-resistant bacteria has become a considerable burden to human health and animal husbandry, and eliminating resistant genotypes from the environment is increasingly challenging. Suspending the use of particular antibiotics has proven ineffective in reducing resistance, because costly resistance mutations are compensated without losing resistance.

The use of bacteriophages to treat bacterial infections (so-called phage therapy) is now being advocated as an alternative to antibiotic therapies.In phage therapy, lytic phages invade specific bacterial strains causing metabolic disruption and cell lysis.

This selective agent, possibly together with an organism's immune response, lowers the bacterial population to levels where it is no longer a danger to the organism. There are many examples of the successful treatment for bacterial infections in experimental and natural settings. For example, lethality of Staphylococcus aureus-induced infections in mice was successfully controlled by the addition of purified phage, such as φMR11.

Whereas selection for antibiotic resistance creates a population of resistant strains that can persist in the environment once compensation for fitness has occurred,in phage therapy populations of bacteria and phages potentially antagonistically coevolve. Here, bacterial populations, if sufficiently genetically variable, will evolve resistance to phage attack.

This, in turn, will select for novel phage genotypes that overcome the resistant phage genotypes.The relevance of coevolution for phage therapy is yet to be established but given evidence that some bacterial pathogens may coevolve with their phage pathogens ,it is important to explore this potentially important mechanism in therapy research.

One possible use of phages for bacterial control is in conjunction with antibiotics. Such combined therapies hold the promise of better control and the slowing of resistance evolution to antibiotics. However, studies devoted to predict the appearance and evolution of resistant populations to both antimicrobial agents are necessary for their rational use when treating bacterial infections. Little is known about the evolutionary effects of both therapies on bacterial populations, either when applied in sequence or simultaneously.

Sequential applications are important to understand, because, for example, the type of mechanism responsible for antibiotic resistance may condition the bacterial response to phage attack and therefore the effectiveness of phage therapy. The simultaneous addition of both selective agents may result in the selection of bacterial variants capable of resisting this complex environment. Resistance may occur either by the use of multipurpose mechanisms or by the convergence to a single optimal variant capable of adapting to both stresses.

In such circumstances, bacterial population persistence will be more likely if large amounts of genetically based variation for adaptation are present, either through standing variation when stresses are introduced or mutations emerging thereafter.

More genetically variable populations will be associated with the presence of hypermutator bacterial strains, and study has shown that coevolution with phages may actually promote mutator emergence (Pal et al. 2007).

Because hypermutator bacteria are abundant in nature, including those associated with infectious diseases,the potential effect of hypermutator genotypes on the bacterial response to single or combined therapies needs to be addressed.

Bacteriophages

Bacteriophages are described as 'phages' for short and, less frequently, as 'bacterial viruses'.

Bacteriophages are the most numerous viruses on Earth, and viruses are more common than bacteria, the most numerous of cellular organisms. Specifically, bacteriophages are the viruses of bacteria, that is, they are sequences of genes (genomes) which move around from bacterium to bacterium while encased within protein shells called capsids, often killing bacteria in the process.

Bacteriophages are hugely important to the ecology and evolution of bacteria, have enormous impacts on the global carbon cycle (which among other things controls whether climates globally warm), represent one promising means by which medicine's current antibiotic crisis – think MRSA – may be overcome.

Phages also contributed greatly to biology's understanding of life in general and especially at the molecular level. They in addition were key to the development of genetic engineering. In short, phages are perhaps the biological world's least appreciated superstars.

Bacteriophages were formally discovered in the mid to late teens of the 20th century, with the first publication coming out in 1915 and then a second in 1917.They were early on speculated to be viral, but their dominant property was an ability to macroscopically "eat" bacterial cultures, specifically by reducing the cloudiness (turbidity) of those cultures.

a consequence of this property, rather than being described as "poisons" (the original meaning of the word "virus"), instead the term "phage" was attached to them, which means to eat or to devour, in Greek. Thus, a bacteriophage is an entity which eats bacteria, though today we know that this descriptor is not perfectly accurate. Nevertheless, phages are capable of macroscopically as well as microscopically destroying populations of bacteria.

Notwithstanding its name, a phage is a virus. A virus is a piece of nucleic acid – RNA or DNA – which is surrounded by a coat that often predominantly consists of protein (called capsid proteins, or capsomeres). The protein capsid's job is protection of the nucleic acid, the genome of the virus, as it moves that genome from infected cell to newly acquired cell.

Cell acquisition is the other job of the capsid, the attachment of the virus to the surface of the cell followed by the movement of the virus' genome into the cell. There virus genes are expressed, giving rise to a diversion of the cell's metabolism (chemical reactions) towards the production of new virus. A successful virus is both effective in finding cells to infect and capable of overcoming cellular or organism-level defenses (collectively, immunity) against virus infection.

A phage specifically is a virus which infects bacteria. In the past few decades microbiologists have come to understand that "bacteria" actually represent a unique taxonomic category, domain Bacteria, which differs in fundamental ways from two other domain-level taxa, domain Archaea and domain Eukarya (domain Eukarya includes us).

Unlike these two latter categories of cellular organisms, whose viruses are called simply viruses, because of the unique history of phage biology it is relatively rare to speak of the viruses of bacteria in those terms. That is, we typically refer to these viruses as bacteriophages, or phages for short. Phages, thus, are the viruses of domain Bacteria. Furthermore, phages are not able to infect members of either domain Archaea or domain Eukarya.

Historical Background

In 1896, Ernest Hanbury Hankin, a British bacteriologist working as the Chemical Examiner and Bacteriologist to the Government of the United Provinces and of the Central Provinces of India, demonstrated that the waters from the Indian rivers Ganga and Yamuna contained a biological principle that destroyed cultures of cholera-inducing bacteria.

This substance could pass through millipore filters, known to be able to retain larger microorganisms such as bacteria. He published his work in French in the Annals of the Pasteur Institute.10 In 1915, while he was studying the growth of vaccinia virus on cell-free agar media, Frederick Twort, a British microbiologist, noted that "pure" cultures of bacteria may be associated with a filter-passing transparent material which may entirely break down bacteria of a culture into granules.

This "filterable agent" was demonstrated in cultures of micrococci isolated from vaccinia: material of some colonies which could not be sub-cultured was able to infect a fresh growth of micrococcus, and this condition could be transmitted to fresh cultures of the microorganism for almost indefinite number of generations. This transparent material, which was found to be unable to grow in the absence of bacteria, was described by Twort as a ferment secreted by the microorganism for some purpose not clear at that time.

Two years after this report, Félix d'Herelle independently described a similar experimental finding, while studying patients suffering or recovering from bacillary dysentery. He isolated from stools of recovering shigellosis patients a so-called "anti-Shiga microbe" by filtering stools that were incubated for 18 h.

This active filtrate, when added either to a culture or an emulsion of the Shiga bacilli, was able to cause arrest of the culture, death and finally lysis of the bacilli. D'Herelle described his discovery as a microbe that was a "veritable" microbe of immunity and an obligate bacteriophage. He also demonstrated the activity of this anti-Shiga microbe by inoculating laboratory animals as a treatment for shigellosis, seeming to confirm the clinical significance of his finding by satisfying at least some of Koch's postulates.

Beyond the actual discussion on origins of d'Herelle himself (some people stating he was born in Paris while others claim he was born in Montreal), the initial controversy was driven mainly by Bordet and his colleague

Gartia at the Institut Pasteur in Brussels. These authors offered competing claims about the exact nature and importance of the fundamental discovery.

While Twort, due to a lack of funds and his enlistment in the Royal Army Medical Corps, did not pursue his research in the same domain, d'Herelle introduced the use of bacteriophages in clinical medicine and published many non-randomized trials from experience all over the world.

He even introduced treatment with intravenous phage for invasive infections, and he summarized all these findings and observations in 1931.heT first published paper on the clinical use of phage, however, was published in Belgium by Bruynoghe and Maisin, who used bacteriophage to treat cutaneous furuncles and carbuncles by injection of staphylococcal-specific phage near the base of the cutaneous boils. They described clear evidence of clinical improvement within 48 h, with reduction in pain, swelling, and fever in treated patients.

At that time, the exact nature of phage had yet to be determined and it remained a matter of active and lively debate. The lack of knowledge of the essential nature of DNA and RNA as the genetic essence of life hampered a fuller understanding about phage biology in the early 20th century.

In 1938 John Northrop still concluded from his own work that bacteriophages were produced by living host by the generation of an inert protein which is changed to the active phage by an auto-catalytic reaction. However, several contributions from other investigators did converge to support d'Herelle's idea that phages were living particles or viruses when replicating in their host cells. In 1928

Wollman assimilated the properties of phages to those of genes,18 an idea already hypothesized by Muller in 1922.

The phenomenon of lysogeny, or the fact that bacteriophages may infect bacteria without the induction of lysis, discovered in 1925 by Bordet and Bail, confirmed the idea that the capacity of reproducing phages within bacteria necessitated the insertion of phage-encoded material into the hereditary units of the host microbe. Frank Macfarlane, an Australian scientist awarded the Nobel Prize in 1960 for his work on immunity, also worked on lysogeny and confirmed the viral nature of phages as well as the nature of its interactions with bacterial hosts.

He also demonstrated that different species of phages did exist.Schlesinger confirmed the biochemical nature of phages made of nucleoproteins allowed the existing theories to join together: phages are viral particles that are made of nucleoproteins.

Finally, the invention of the electron microscope (EM) allowed Helmut Ruska, a German doctor, to first describe round particles as well as "sperm-shaped" particles from a phage suspension adhering to a bacterial membrane.Two years later, he summarized his principal research into the nature and biology of bacteriophages in his thesis work.

One year after the first description of phages with EM, Luria and Anderson, in Camden, New Jersey, visualized different types of phages and described their common structure: a non-homogeneous round head with a much thinner tail, giving the peculiar sperm-like appearance.They also described the various stages of bacteria lysis: adsorption which increases with time, extensive bacterial damage and appearance of a large number of newly formed bacteriophages.

While research on phage was never abandoned in the former USSR, with the development of the Eliava Institute in Tbilissi, Georgia, and some other countries such as Poland (and its well-known Hirsfeld Institute in Wroclaw), the English literature rediscovered phage therapy in animals in the 1980s and human experiments started in the 2000s, with the first phase I randomized trial in the US published in 2009.

In August 2004, the so-called Phage Summit was held in Key Biscayne, Florida, and more than 350 conferees attended this first major international gathering in decades devoted to phage biology, demonstrating the explosive resurgence of interest in this field.Overall, the phage literature has become one of the most expansive topics, rendering bacteriophages as one of the best studied microbes known to science. In 1958 and 1967, Raettig published 2 bibliographies, covering about 358 references.

In 2012, Ackerman analyzed 30 000 phage publications published between 1965 and 2010.34 The names of first authors represent 40 linguistic domains or geographic areas and at least 70 languages, leading to the conclusion that phage particles are studied all over the world (even if English and German languages predominate).

What Are Phages?

Viruses are very diverse, in part because there are many ways that a cell can be hijacked to produce more viruses, and also because there are many ways that cells can block virus infections. Thus, viruses probably are subject to what is known as frequency-dependent selection for diversity. Phages are no exception.

Like viruses in general, phages vary in terms of the basic structure of their genomes (their nucleic acid) as well as the structure of their proteinaceous capsids, and even can have lipids (fat-like molecules) in their coats (as do many animal viruses).

In short, phages can have DNA or RNA genomes (unlike cellular organisms whose genomes uniformly consist of DNA), they can infect in ways that kill their hosts or in ways which do not (just like, for example, animal viruses), and they can take on a variety of morphologies, some relatively simple, and some quite complex.

It is these morphologies which are the most recognizable feature of phages. In particular, phages can be differentiated into those which possess substantial appendages called tails and those which do not. The tail is invariably attached to a head – at least among functional phages – and together they form the "lunar lander"-looking structure that nearly universally says "virus", even to many who have little idea of what a virus in fact is.

It is within the head, which takes on a geometrical shape called a polyhedron (more strictly, an icosahedron), that the DNA is found, and it is through the tail that the DNA is delivered to an unsuspecting bacterium.

Alternatively, phages that possess unusual genomes, consisting in some cases of either

RNA or only half of the DNA double helix, or which possess lipids in their capids, to at least a first approximation are both not and never tailed. To the extent we can describe viruses as organisms, the tailed phages in fact appear to be the most numerous category of organisms on Earth.

The primary phage task is the infection of bacteria, production of new phages, and the release of those phages from the infected bacterium. For tailed phages that release consists of lysis, which is the destruction of the outer portion of the bacterium so that the phage virions (virus particles) that form inside of the infected cell can reach the outside (surfaces) of new cells to infect.

This lysis can be viewed as a form of decay, that is, lysis is one means of converting bacteria into soluble nutrients which are then available to other organisms, where these other organisms to a large extent consist of other bacteria.

Alternatively, phages, in a process called transduction, can fail to lyse a bacterium, following infection, but instead carry new genes into that bacterium, in some cases converting otherwise benign bacteria into potential pathogens. Ongoingly, all around us, and even inside of us, phages affect bacteria in ways that can have profound effects on the world around us.

What are phages good for?

Phages play important roles in the ecology and evolution of bacteria. In fact, bacteria probably wouldn't be bacteria, at least as they exist today, without phages moving their DNA among themselves (phage-mediated DNA transduction) or phage-mediated diversification of their bacterial prey (frequency-dependent selection for more diverse bacteria-encoded anti-phage mechanisms along with the elimination of too successful bacteria, i.e., so-called "Killing the winner").

Much of what goes on between phages and bacteria, however, represents something of an ecological background, that is, it is simply what happens out there in the nature. Alternatively, the ability of phages to move DNA around, as noted, can give rise to bacterial pathogens, and indeed a number of phages actually encode toxins which can make us sick, including the toxins (actually "exotoxins") associated with the bacteria responsible for cholera, diphtheria, and even E. coli O157:H7, the so-called hamburger E. coli .

The term "Antitoxin" in its original popularization in fact was short for "antidiphtheria toxin" where diphtheria toxin is the proximate cause of diphtheria – that is, the bacterium without this toxin will not cause diphtheria – but, in fact, diphtheria toxin is a expressed from a phage gene.

Given this apparent infamy, can we still speak of phages as, well, good? The answer seems to in fact be yes for at least four technologies. First, research on phages both underlies and continues to provide important tools for the molecular analysis of life, a key component of modern biomedical research (think biotech industry).

Second, phages play important roles in the monitoring of environmental quality, especially by serving as surrogates for human viruses, both as indicators of fecal contamination and as models for virus dissemination especially in association with water. Third, phages have and continue to play important roles in the identification, classification, characterization, and detection of especially pathogenic bacteria. Lastly, phages are capable of killing both nuisance and pathogenic bacteria, in the guise of so-called phage therapy.

Types of Phages and Phage Biology

More than 6000 different bacteriophages have been discovered and described morphologically, including 6196 bacterial and 88 archeal viruses. The vast majority of these viruses are tailed while a small proportion are polyhedral, filamentous or pleomorphic.

They may be classified according to their morphology, their genetic content (DNA vs. RNA), their specific host (for instance the staphylococcal phage family, the Pseudomonas phage family, and so on), the place where they live (marine virus vs. other habitats), and their life cycle. Evolving classification formats have been proposed over time and abbreviations for these viruses were proposed by Fauquet and Pringle in 2000.

As obligatory intracellular parasite of a bacterial cell, phages display different life cycles within the bacterial host: lytic, lysogenic, pseudo-lysogenic, and chronic infection. For phage therapy, the main interest has focused upon lytic phages, mainly represented in 3 families of the Caudovirales order: the Myoviridae, the Siphoviridae and the Podoviridae.

There are also some reports on cubic phages and filamentous phages applications.General description of those phages may be summarized as follows: the genetic material is contained in a protein shell or capsid which has a form of an icosahedron; this head is connected through a collar to the tail which may be contractile or not and whose distal extremity is in contact with tail fibers with tips that recognize attachment sites on receptors of the bacterial cell surface.

Whatever the type of cycle of a phage life, the first step is the attachment to receptors of the bacterial cell wall before phages may enter the bacteria. This specific process influences the spectrum of the possible phage-bacteria interactions. For instance, bacteriophage λ interacts only with the LamB receptor of E. coli. Spatiotemporal dynamics have demonstrated this event to be of major importance for successful bacterial invasion.

Some phages also are able to synthesize specific enzymes (such as hydrolases or polysaccharidases and polysaccharide lyases) able at degrading exopolysaccharide structure capsules, before they may interact with their specific receptor. This is the case for some phages interacting with strains of E. coli, V. cholerae, P. aeruginosa, E. agglomerans, and P. putida. These enzymes are of potential interest for their therapeutic implications and are in pre-clinical development at present.

Upon binding to its specific receptor, phages induce a pore in the bacterial cell wall and inject its DNA into the cell, while the viral capsid remains outside of the bacteria. This is followed by the expression of phage early genes, which, in the case of lytic phages, redirects the bacterial synthetic machinery to the reproduction of viral nucleic acids and proteins.

Assembly and packing of phages is then observed before bacterial cell lysis and release of phage progeny occur. Phages' late enzymes such as lysins, holins, and murein synthesis inhibitors are then employed for the virion burst in the extracellular environment. The number of viral particles released, or burst size, greatly varies according to the phage, the state of the bacteria host, and other environmental factors such as nutritive components surrounding the host.

In the lysogenic cycle, the so-called temperate phages insert their genetic content (the prophage) in the chromosomes of the bacteria, where it remains silent for extended periods and is replicated as part of the bacterial chromosome. Hence, there is no self-replication.

This prophage DNA is vertically transmitted along with the whole bacterial genome to its progeny until the lytic cycle is induced.During induction lysogenic phage can on occasion transfer host genetic material adjacent to its insertion site on the chromosome from one bacterium to another, a phenomenon called transduction.

Actually, the fact that phages are of major importance for bacterial genome evolution is a concept known for years, and Brussow even described bacteriophages as agents for lateral gene transfer.This process can promote the transfer of genes that are of selective advantage for bacterial host including antibiotic resistance genes; however, the same process could be exploited therapeutically by using phage to transfer genes rendering bacteria more susceptible to some antibiotics.

Indeed, by targeting the mechanisms of DNA repair with the injection of a specific gene which led to the overexpression of a protein that inhibits this system, Lu and Collins demonstrated, in vitro, an increased susceptibility of E. coli to antibiotics.Gene insertion was achieved through a specific, and modified, bacteriophage M13. Interestingly, they also used the same technique in mice, intraperitoneally infected with E. coli.

Survival was increased in mice concomitantly treated with antibiotics and modified phages. This approach was found by other authors to be similar to the general approach of phage therapy that leads to direct killing of bacteria.

Another approach consists in reversing the pathogen drug resistance by injecting specific genes for a sensitizing cassette conferring susceptibility in a dominant fashion. This was recently demonstrated by Edgar and colleagues who were able to render resistant bacteria susceptible to streptomycin and nalidixic acid.Finally, the chronic infection occurs when the bacteria is infected by lysogenic phage that subsequently mutates and loses the capacity to induce a lytic replication cycle. The phage DNA becomes a new part of the bacterial chromosome and becomes a long-term prophage sequence.

Why We Need Phage Therapy

Over the 2 or 3 last decades, the widespread emergence and spread of antibiotic-resistant bacteria around the world has become a major therapeutic challenge.For instance, MRSA infections in the US were reported with an incidence of about 100 000 serious infections in 2005, contributing to 20 000 deaths.

The limited therapeutic options remaining to treat major multi-drug resistant (MDR) bacteria, known by the acronym as the ESKAPE pathogens (for Enterococcus faecium, Staphylococcus aureus, Klebsiella pneumoniae, Acinetobacter baumannii, Pseudomonas aeruginosa, and Enterobacter spp.), has now become a looming healthcare crisis in many ICUs worldwide.Treating patients with MDR pathogens has been demonstrated by Morales et al. to increase the total cost of care and to prolong hospital length of stay.

An ethical imperative exists throughout the health care professions to do all we can to preserve the efficacy of antibiotics and recognize that this precious resource is being squandered by often unnecessary and inappropriate antibiotic use, promoting the acquisition and dissemination of antibiotic resistance genes.

Antibiotic drug resistance is now recognized as a health care emergency and appeals for the development of novel means to combat it have been voiced by many; however, antibiotics are developed on the basis of free market criteria, rather than on the basis of direct benefit to the public.However, despite the call for the development of new antibiotics in the European Union (EU) and in the United

States (US), there is dearth of new antibiotics in the developmental pipeline.

An entirely novel, non-antibiotic approach to treat bacterial pathogens is certainly needed. The re-deployment of phage therapy could become a welcome alternative to antimicrobial chemotherapy in this period of progressive spread of MDR bacterial pathogens with a paucity of new antibiotic to combat these pathogens.

Furthermore, the need for phage applications certainly exceeds its use in human infections. Indeed the use of bacteriophages has been described in various situations including (but not limited to): food safety,agriculture, veterinary applications,industry, and clinical diagnostic application such as detection and typing of bacteria in human infection.

Potential Advantages of Phage Therapy

Bacteriophages are natural antibacterials able to regulate bacterial populations by the induction of bacterial lysis. They are active against gram-positive, as well as gram-negative bacteria, including MDR pathogens. Indeed, as mechanism of action phage lysis is totally different from antibiotics, retaining activity against bacteria exhibiting multiple mechanisms of antibiotic resistance.

Because of its specificity, phage therapy has a narrow antibacterial spectrum with an effect limited to one single species or in some cases a single strain within a species. This limits the "pressure" and the heavy collateral damage done to bystander, non-targeted bacteria from antibiotics. The entire microbiome of the patient is altered by antibiotics, not just the intended target pathogen.

In contrast, Chibani-Chennoufi et al. demonstrated little impact on the gut microbiota in mice after oral administration of phage therapy directed against E. coli. Preservation of much of the existing microbiome during phage therapy has been confirmed in careful microbial surveys in adult healthy volunteers who ingested a 9-phage cocktail. Phage therapy also avoids the potential overgrowth of secondary pathogens.

Since large, randomized, controlled trials are lacking at the present time, it is difficult to evaluate side effects and their potential impact. Based on the reports gained from Poland and the former Soviet Union, phage therapy seems to be without significant adverse effects; the fact that bacteriophages interact with bacterial cells only and do not interfere with mammalian cells probably could potentially explain this lack of deleterious side effects.

Underreporting could be another explanation. However, the excellent tolerability of phage treatment has been demonstrated in preclinical studies in various animal models and in several observational studies in patients and healthy human volunteers There is a wide distribution of phages upon systemic administration, including the ability to penetrate the blood brain barrier, allowing these agents to be used in case of central nervous system infections.Interestingly, at least some phages also display the capacity to disrupt bacterial biofilms.

Phage therapy may have an impact on the inflammatory response to infection. In patients presenting with various long-term suppurative infection, TNFα release, in vivo and in vitro upon stimulation with LPS, was attenuated based upon the initial pattern of serum TNFα level.

Release of IL-6 was only significantly reduced in vivo.-reactive protein and white blood cell count were initially not affected in this patient population while it significantly decreased between day 9 and day 32 in 37 patients given oral phage therapy for osteomyelitis, prosthetic joint infection, skin and soft tissue infections, and, in one case, lung infection.

This was an observational study without a control group and therefore should be cautiously interpreted. In a more recent observation, CRP was only affected in patients whose initial CRP serum level was above 10 mg/dl. White blood cells may also be affected by phage therapy: increased neutrophil precursors and decreased phagocytic index for Staphylococcus aureus was observed in patients after 3 weeks and 3 mo of therapy, as compared with healthy donors.A large review of the alteration of immune responses with phage therapy has recently been published.

Finally, the economic aspects of phage therapy look promising. Despite the fact that the duration of treatment was significantly prolonged, the cost of phage therapy was lower than conventional antibiotic treatment as it was demonstrated in 6 patients presenting with various staphylococcal infections including methicillin resistant Staphylococcus aureus.80

Above all, the fact that bacteriophages could have an improved efficacy as compared with antibiotics provides the greatest hope for the future. Smith and colleagues first demonstrated this finding in the early 1980s when they induced a lethal E. coli infection in mice using a highly virulent strain expressing a K1 polysaccharide capsule.One single intramuscular dose of anti-K1 phage was as effective as multiple streptomycin injections, and was superior to multiple intramuscular doses of tetracycline, ampicillin, chloramphenicol, or trimethoprim in curing the animals. To our knowledge, this observation has never been confirmed in human infection.

Actually, the optimal dose, route of administration, frequency, and duration of treatment still need to be defined before widespread clinical trials are contemplated.

The major disadvantage of phage therapy is the need to rapidly determine the precise etiological microorganism causing infection with accuracy. The exquisite specificity of phage therapy against specific pathogens is a major advantage, but also a liability. A clinical sample has to be isolated and cultured, using standard microbiology diagnostic procedures, to identify the pathogen before a specific bacteriophage solution may be defined and later on administered to the patient.

Innovations in rapid bacterial diagnosis with genomic methods or the use of mass spectroscopy might help. Nonetheless, this is a time consuming process in most clinical microbiology laboratories and in resource-limited health care settings.

This problem could potentially be solved with the use of ready to use phage "cocktails". Selection of potent phages from an available collection after phage typing of the isolated bacteria defines the so-called composed phage cocktail treatment.

Finally, when no active, existing phage preparation is present against a severe pathogen, it can be isolated directly from the environment before it is prepared for application. For instance, in the recent outbreak of E. coli O104:H4 in Germany, active lytic phages were found in the collection of the Eliava Institute (Georgia) as well as in the wastewater of the Brussels Military Hospital in Belgium.

The choice of bacteriophage for therapy is limited to lytic phages. Indeed, lysogenic phages will induce delayed lysis, preventing application of those phages in an acute infection. Although standardized methods to generate phage cocktails do exist, there are no clear official guidelines.Virion stability in terms of their susceptibility to various external and physical factors has recently been reviewed and could account for some difficulties in preparing stable solutions.

Another concern of phage therapy is the potential ability of bacteriophages to transfer the DNA from a bacterium to another. This transfer of genetic material, or transduction, could be responsible for the transfer of pathogenicity determinants and virulence factors, leading to the development of a new microbe or even more resistant bacteria.Therefore, the use of phages unable to package extra host DNA or phages that use the host DNA to synthesize its own DNA would be preferred. This technique has already been successfully applied in phage therapy.

The genome of many phages has been unraveled and each month, there are reports on newly identified gene sequences. However, we are far from having sequenced the gene of each type of phages88 and the function of many of these genes is still unknown. For instance, the ORFan genes found in some phages have no similarity to any other gene in the gene database. The role of those genes in the potential to promote deleterious side effects has still to be elucidated.

At the end of its antibacterial action, lytic phages induce the lysis of bacteria, liberating various bacterial substances such as endotoxin (LPS) from gram-negative bacteria. This may account for several side effects on the host such as the development of an inflammatory cascade leading to multiple organ failure. However, this potential issue applies to currently available rapidly bactericidal antibiotics.

Since they are viruses, bacteriophages may be seen by the immune system of the patient as a potential invader and may therefore rapidly be eliminated from the systemic circulation by reticulo-endothelial system clearance before they are accumulated in the spleen or the liver, or, they may be inactivated by the adaptive immune defense mechanisms.91 This could lead to a decreased efficacy in case of prolonged or repeated applications.

Finally, the development of resistance mechanisms by the bacterial host, resulting either from mutation and selection or by temperate phage acquisition, could lead to a decreased efficacy of phages. There are at least 4 mechanisms that may be involved in bacterial resistance to a specific phage. Loss or lack of receptor, structural modification and, or masking of the receptor will prevent phage adsorption to the bacteria and prevent further ability to generate new phages.

Loss of receptor may occur when cell surface composition is changed, as was demonstrated for Bordetella spp.Structural modification has been noticed for E. coli protein TraT which modifies the conformation of the Outer-Membrane Protein A (OmpA), the receptor for T-even-like phages.

Secretion of various molecules (such as exopolysaccharide by Pseudomonas spp. or glycoconjugates by Enterobacteriacae) may mask the receptor, but phages may counteract this by the selection of a new receptor or by secreting exopolysaccharide degrading enzyme.

The other mechanisms of resistance include the prevention of phage DNA integration by superinfection exclusion system (Sie), degradation of phage DNA by Restriction-Modification defense system or by Clustered Regularly Interspaced Short Palindromic Repeats (CRISPR), and the blocking of phage replication, transcription, translation, or virions assembly by Abortive Infection system.

Fortunately, thus far the frequency of resistance in vivo during phage therapy is reportedly low, as opposed to the observed in vitro resistance analyses. Furthermore, isolation of novel active phages from the environment or progressive isolation of "adapted" phages could provide a new possibility for treatment.

In most countries, phage therapy is not covered by public health insurance, a potential financial problem for some patients. Some exceptions do exist. Switzerland authorities decided to reimburse complementary medicine for a period of 6 years, while efficacy is evaluated95 and the president of the city of Wroclaw (where the Hirszfeld Institute is located), Poland, has established a program covering the costs of phage therapy for the residents of the city; 2 examples to be followed according to Myedzybrodzki.

Since bacterial viruses are currently not recognized as medicinal products, current European pharmacological regulations, definitions and standards are not adequately adapted to phage preparations.Therefore, a Belgian Research group and some members of the Pasteur Institute in Paris, developed the P.H.A.G.E. an international non-profit organization, with the aim to develop a specific framework for the use of bacteriophages.

Regulatory clearance remains another hurdle. In addition to the inherent safety concern, neither the US Food and Drug Administration nor the European Medicines Agency has an approval process in place that can easily accommodate the ever-changing combina-tions of phages that companies need to develop to stay one step ahead of evolving MDR bacteria.

Already Described Human Applications

The first report on the use of bacteriophage in humans described its efficacy in staphylococcal skin furuncles16 and d'Herelle summarized all his clinical work in 1931. There were a large amount of publications in the 1930s and a full monograph of the journal La Médicine covered phage applications in human disease.

It described the treatment of typhoid fever, Shigella and Salmonella spp.-related colitis, peritonitis, skin infections, surgical infections (mainly abscesses of various locations), septicemia, urinary tract infections, and otolaryngology infections (external otitis and nasal furuncles).

However, as already described, the enthusiasm for phage therapy declined in the western countries in the 1930s because of the questions regarding scientific rigor in testing phage therapy in the reports by Eaton and colleagues and also as a consequence of the discovery and the ease of use of antibiotics.

The use of bacteriophages continued in the eastern countries and large number of reports were published over time, mainly in Poland and Georgia (former USSR). The use of non-English literature (mainly Russian and Polish) probably explain the fact those reports were confined to the country of origin of the authors.

A summary of this literature have been published by various authors more recently,showing extensive experience for some authors with several hundred treated patients.We, however, have to note that most of the published data are from non-randomized, uncontrolled trials.

Indeed, the first phase I randomized controlled trial conducted in the United States was published in 2009.[31] It evaluated the safety of a cocktail of phages directed against E. coli, S. aureus, and Pseudomonas aeruginosa in 42 patients with chronic venous leg ulcers.

study was not powered to detect any positive outcome such as rate or frequency of healing but the authors did not find any adverse event related to the treatment. Another randomized trial was conducted in the UK and studied the efficacy of one application of a solution containing 6 bacteriophages in the ears of patients suffering chronic Pseudomonas aeruginosa-related otitis.

The colony counts of P. aeruginosa significantly decreased in the treated group in this well done, double-blind, placebo-controlled study while various subjective clinical indicators improved in those patients. Indeed, patients reported lower intensity of symptoms such as discomfort, itching, wetness, and unpleasant odor.

Likewise, physicians in charge of the patients (and blinded to the assigned treatment) reported decreased clinical observations such as erythema/inflammation, ulceration/granulation/polyps, and odor. There were no reported adverse reactions.

A small phase I study of 9 patients treated at the Burn Wound Centre of the Queen Astrid Military Hospital, Brussels, Belgium, was recently performed.110 Patients were locally treated with the BFC-1 phage cocktail containing 3 lytic phages: a Myovirus, a Podovirus against Pseudomonas aeruginosa, and a Myovirus directed against Staphylococcus aureus.

A large burned section was exposed to a single spray application while a distant portion of the wound served as control. While complete results are yet to be published, there was no safety issue reported.

Finally, a randomized controlled trial confirmed the safety of an orally administered phage solution in healthy non-infected patients.

Phage Therapy

Phage therapy is the application of phages that can kill bacteria to reduce in number or eliminate those bacteria. Phage therapy has at least four advantages over conventional antibiotic therapy.First, relatively rare encoding of exotoxins aside, phage virions are inherently safe, consisting of just benign proteins and DNA, and therefore display a larger therapeutic window, the difference between their toxic dose and their therapeutic dose.

Vancomycin, typically described as an antibiotic of last resort, instead displays a very small therapeutic window, meaning that, unlike with phages, it is relatively difficult to avoid adverse effects.

Second, phages are fairly narrow in their spectrum of activity, meaning that with phage treatment it is possible to kill bacterial pathogens while avoiding the harming of normal flora bacteria, that is, our good bacteria.

Because of this narrow spectrum of activity, with phage treatment superinfections are must less likely (contrast antibiotic-associated "C-Diff" or vaginal yeast superinfections), plus phages may be employed prophylactically with little fear of adversely affecting patients.

The third advantage of phages is that they often are capable of replicating to higher densities in situ, that is, within their target environment, such as our bodies. This may allow phages to penetrate further into bacterial infections, such as those which have formed biofilms.

It also eases dosing concerns, as above, though in the other direction, that is, in addition to delivering too high phage doses being less of a concern (in comparison to many antibiotics), in fact delivering too low phage doses, at least under certain circumstances, also can be less of a concern since phages reaching bacteria will tend to replicate. This replication produces locally high densities of phages which, in turn, can lead to bacterial demise.

Fourth, and finally, phages are hugely numerous and hugely diverse. Therefore the "discovery" of novel phages with novel activities (especially novel spectra of activity) is very simple, often involving little more than a short trip down to a local sewage treatment plant for a sampling of untreated influent (don't worry, not only is this a standard procedure in microbiology, but the phages are fully separated from the rest of the components of sewage well before they are turned into a product).

With modern sequencing technology along with bioinformatics (the analysis of the genes of organisms) even full phage genetic characterization can be a relatively trivial endeavor.

Phages are natural, ubiquitous, in most circumstances harmless, and relatively easy to thoroughly characterize. They have the useful property of being able to kill bacteria that we don't like or want, plus have been used in this regard for going on one-hundred years. With the potential to become a technology of first resort in the humanity's ongoing battle against infectious disease, it is just a matter of time before the term "phage" becomes a household word.

Pros and Cons of Phage Therapy

Phages can be bactericidal, can increase in number over the course of treatment, tend to only minimally disrupt normal flora, are equally effective against antibiotic-sensitive and antibiotic-resistant bacteria, often are easily discovered, seem to be capable of disrupting bacterial biofilms, and can have low inherent toxicities.

In addition to these assets, we consider aspects of phage therapy that can contribute to its safety, economics, or convenience, but in ways that are perhaps less essential to the phage potential to combat bacteria.

For example, autonomous phage transfer between animals during veterinary application could provide convenience or economic advantages by decreasing the need for repeated phage application, but is not necessarily crucial to therapeutic success. We also consider possible disadvantages to phage use as antibacterial agents. These "Cons," however, tend to be relatively minor.

Introduced in the early 1900s,1 phage therapy is the application of bacteria-specific viruses (phages) to combat uncontrolled and undesired bacteria such as those associated with infectious disease. In reviews of phage therapy3 authors commonly list advantages of employing phages as antibacterials. These lists can be used as talking points of why, in this age of epidemic antibiotic resistance, phage therapy should not be overlooked.

Major Advantages of Phage Therapy

Advantages of phage therapy over the use of chemical antibiotics can be framed in terms of phage properties. In this section we consider those properties that, in our opinion, can contribute substantially to phage therapy utility.

Bactericidal agents

Bacteria that have been successfully infected by obligately lytic phages are unable to regain their viability. By contrast, certain antibiotics are bacteriostatic, such as tetracycline, and as a consequence may more readily permit bacterial evolution towards resistance.

Auto "dosing".

Phages during the bacterial-killing process are capable of increasing in number specifically where hosts are located,though with some limitations such as dependence on relatively high bacterial densities.We call this auto "dosing" because the phages themselves contribute to establishing the phage dose.

Low inherent toxicity.

Since phages consist mostly of nucleic acids and proteins, they are inherently nontoxic.However, phages can interact with immune systems, at least potentially resulting in harmful immune responses, though there is little evidence that this actually is a concern during phage treatment.

Nonetheless, it can be imperative for certain phage therapy protocols to use highly purified phage preparations8 to prevent anaphylactic responses to bacterial components, such as the endotoxins that can be found in crude phage lysates.Phages similarly can release bacterial components while killing bacteria in situ, a property associated with lysis that also can result from the application of cell-wall disrupting antibiotics.

Minimal disruption of normal flora.

Owing to their host specificity—which can range from an ability to infect only a few strains of a bacterial species to, more rarely, a capacity to infect more than one relatively closely related bacterial genus—phages only minimally impact health-protecting normal flora bacteria.By contrast, many chemical antibiotics, which tend to have broader spectrums of activity, are prone to inducing superinfections, such as antibiotic-associated Clostridium difficile colitis or Candida albicans yeast infections.The historical bias towards developing only broader spectrum antibiotics, however, may be changing.

Narrower potential for inducing resistance.

The relatively narrow host range exhibited by most phages limits the number of bacterial types with which selection for specific phage-resistance mechanisms can occur. This contrasts with the substantial fraction of bacteria that can be affected by most chemical antibiotics. In addition, some mutations to resistance negatively impact bacterial fitness or virulence due to loss of pathogenicity-related phage receptors.

Lack of cross-resistance with antibiotics.

Because phages infect and kill using mechanisms that differ from those of antibiotics, specific antibiotic resistance mechanisms do not translate into mechanisms of phage resistance. Phages consequently can be readily employed to treat antibiotic-resistant infections such as against multi-drug-resistance Staphylococcus aureus.

Rapid discovery.

Phages against many pathogenic bacteria are easily discovered, often from sewage and other waste materials that contain high bacterial concentrations. Isolation can be more technically demanding, however, if host bacteria themselves are difficult to culture and bacteria may differ in terms of the number of phage types to which they are susceptible Unlike antibiotics, which can be toxic, phages that display little or no toxicity can be isolated against most target bacteria.

Formulation and application versatility.

Phages, like antibiotics, can be versatile in terms of formulation development, such as being combined with certain antibiotics.They are also versatile in application form, as liquids, creams, impregnated into solids, etc., in addition to being suitable for most routes of administration. Different phages furthermore can be mixed as cocktails to broaden their properties, typically resulting in a collectively greater antibacterial spectrum of activity.

Biofilm clearance.

Biofilms tend to be substantially more resistant to antibiotics than planktonic bacteria. Phages, however, have a demonstrated ability to clear at least some biofilms, perhaps owing to a potential to actively penetrate their way into biofilms by lysing one bacterial layer at a time, or due to the display of biofilm exopolymer-degrading depolymerases.

Additional Advantages of Phage Therapy

The following advantages associated with the use of phages as antibacterials have possible safety-, economic-, or convenience-enhancing virtues but are not essential to phage antibacterial use.

Single dose potential.

Applying phages in only a single dose takes advantage of the phage potential to replicate and thereby achieve 'active' therapy, i.e., significant phage amplification via auto "dosing" that results in greater bacterial kiling.Achieving efficacy following only a single dose, or far less frequent dosing, is an obvious convenience, though in many or most instances a single dosage of phages should not be expected, a priori, to be sufficient to achieve desired efficacy.

Possible transfer of phages between subjects.

This is essentially cross-infection of phages from treated subjects or environments to untreated subjects. This could be useful in some agricultural applications.

Capacity for low-dosage use.

The ability of phages to increase in density in situ, given sufficient bacterial densities, could potentially reduce treatment costs by reducing phage doses required to achieve efficacy.Application of phages in low doses may also improve product safety, since phages will only increase in density if they are actively killing bacteria and do not otherwise linger long within the body.

Avoiding phage application at higher doses for safety reasons, however, has utility only if phage application at higher doses is not safe, but there is little evidence suggesting that higher versus lower phage doses may be associated with increases in side effects, especially when using purified phage preparations.

Single hit kinetics.

Unlike chemical antibiotics, only a single phage is needed to kill a single bacterium. Often fewer "units" of phages therefore are required per treatment, though high multiplicities of phage adsorption to bacteria are still necessary to substantially reduce target bacterial densities.

Low environmental impact.

Because they are composed predominantly of nucleic acids and proteins,3 and possess relatively narrow host ranges,discarded therapeutic phages, unlike broad-spectrum chemical antibiotics, will at worst have an impact on only a small subset of environmental bacteria. Phages not adapted to degradative environmental factors, such as sunlight, desiccation, or temperature extremes, also can be rapidly inactivated.

Phages are not antibiotics.

There are a number of non-essential uses of antibiotics that contribute to bacterial evolution of resistance: antibiotic treatment of animal or plant diseases, antibiotic use to increase food-animal growth rates, and over- or improper use of antibiotics to treat human diseases. In addition, there is concern about antibiotic contamination of foods (e.g., milk) as well as of downstream environments such as from sewage effluent. Since phages do not contribute to antibiotic resistance, using phages to replace antibiotics could help extend the clinical utility of conventional antibiotics.

Phages are natural products.

Public resistance to laboratory-synthesized drugs or genetically modified organisms should not apply to non-engineered phage products as they are natural components of environments.

Relatively low cost.

The production of phages predominately involves a combination of host growth and subsequent purification.While the cost of host growth varies depending upon bacterial species, the cost of phage purification appears to be coming down as technology improves.Generally these costs of phage production, per unit, are not out of line with the costs of pharmaceutical production while the costs of discovery (isolation) and characterization can be relatively low.

Potential Disadvantages

Concerns about using phages as antibacterial agents can be distinguished into four categories:

(1) phage selection,

(2) phage host-range limitations,

(3) the "uniqueness" of phages as pharmaceuticals, and

(4) unfamiliarity with phages.

Not all phages make for good therapeutics.

Good therapeutic phages should have a high potential to reach and then kill bacteria in combination with a low potential to otherwise negatively modify the environments to which they are applied. These characteristics can be reasonably assured so long as phages are obligately lytic, stable under typical storage conditions and temperatures, subject to appropriate efficacy and safety studies, and, ideally, fully sequenced to confirm the absence of undesirable genes such as toxins.

Note that a phage that is "obligately lytic" we define as not temperate and released from infected cells via lysis, that is, unable to display lysogeny and not released chronically. The use of temperate phages as therapeutics is problematic due to a combination of display of superinfection immunity,which converts phage-sensitive bacteria into insensitive ones, and the encoding of bacterial virulence factors, including bacterial toxins.

In addition to avoiding temperate or toxin-carrying phages, the aim of phage characterization is to exclude as therapeutics those phages that display poor killing potential against target bacteria. Such low "virulence" can be due to poor adsorption properties, low potential to evade bacterial defenses, or poor replication characteristics.

Also less desirable for therapeutics are those phages that display poor pharmacokinetics, that is, poor absorption, distribution, and survival in situ. Ideally phages should also display a low potential to transfer bacterial genes between bacteria (transduction).

Phage characterization additionally can include virion morphology (via electron microscopy), protein profiles, or genotype characterization other than via full-genome sequencing (e.g., PFGE profiles of restriction digested genomes), etc., though the costs associated with exhaustive phage characterization prior to phage use can be prohibitive.

The general aim, therefore, should be to identify those phages that display good primary pharmacodynamics (that is, antibacterial virulence), minimal secondary pharmacodynamics (low potential to do harm to patients), and good pharmacokinetics (an ability to reach target bacteria in situ).

Phages that do not adequately meet these criteria should in most circumstances not be employed as therapeutics. Minimally this should entail avoiding temperate phages and, ideally, full genome sequencing should be used to rule out virulence-factor carriage.

The problem of narrow host range.

No antimicrobials displaying selective toxicity will affect all possible microbial targets. Typically the narrowness of phage host ranges—a few strains, a few species, or much rarer, a few genera of bacteria—will at a minimum place limitations on presumptive treatment, i.e., treatment courses that begin prior to the identification of the pathogen's susceptibility to antibacterials such as to specific phages.

However, as phages can often be employed in combination with other antibacterial agents, including other phages (so-called phage cocktails), the lytic spectrum of phage products can be much broader than the spectrum of activity of individual phage types.Even broadly acting phage cocktails are normally more selective in their spectrum of activity than typical 'narrow-spectrum' antibiotics, a property that can be viewed as an additional advantage of phage therapy.

Phages are not unique pharmaceuticals...

Phages as pharmaceuticals are protein-based, live-biological agents that can potentially interact with the body's immune system, can actively replicate, and can even evolve during manufacture or use, but are far from unique in these regards.

For example, many protein-based pharmaceuticals can stimulate immune systems, antibiotics that lyse bacteria will release bacterial toxins in situ, and live-attenuated vaccines both actively replicate and evolve including within the context of infecting body tissues. Protein-based drugs, chemical antibiotics, and whole vaccines have previously been approved for use despite these various properties. It therefore stands to reason that phage-based pharmaceuticals should not be disqualified for possessing similar attributes.

Phage Therapy and Antibiotics

Antibiotics are small molecules that are used to cures severe infection caused by pathogenic bacteria. Antibiotics kill or stop bacterial growth by several ways, as they disrupt bacterial cell wall, plasma membrane, stop DNA replication, transcription, and protein synthesis. There are mainly two types of antibiotics namely broad-spectrum antibiotics that affect a wide range of bacteria and narrow spectrum antibiotics that affect only one or a few type of bacteria.

The mode of action of different antibiotics is different depending on chemical nature of antibiotics and bacterial species. Due to excessive use many bacteria have developed resistance to many antibiotics and such bacteria referred as Multi Drug Resistant bacteria. For the treatment of infections caused by these MDR bacterial strains needs to develop a novel alternative antimicrobial agents.

Bacteriophage is the virus that infects and kills the bacteria and may be used as an alternative antimicrobial therapy[1]. Bacteriophages are highly specific means they infect only one or a few types of bacteria and non-toxic to human, animals and plants. Bacteriophage therapy is superior to antibiotics because bacteriophage is the only unique class of antimicrobials whose titer increases during the course of therapy that leads to increase in efficacy.

Therefore, in this chapter we are highlighting the bacteriophages therapy to reconsidered as an approach to combat with increasing drug resistance among pathogenic bacteria.

One of the greatest scientific achievements of the twentieth century was the development and mass production of antibiotics, to cope with increasing incidences of bacterial infections. Over past 60 years antibiotic become most reliable and widely used prescriptions against bacterial diseases. But more frequent and uncontrolled use of this miracle cure, the bacteria start getting resistance against many established antibiotics.

This inherent feature of bacteria to develop resistance posed a serious threat to our chemical shield that has been increasingly leaked. World Health Organization (WHO) warned that "the world is on the brink of losing these miracle cures -the antibiotics" and that "in the absence of urgent corrective and protective actions, the world is heading toward a post-antibiotic era, in which many common infections will no longer have a cure and, once again, kill unabated".

Thus it seems unrealistic to depend entirely on antibiotics against bacterial threats, and even the most effective antibiotics have also detrimental effects on endogenous gut microbiome which plays a vital role in human digestion and nutrition. Additionally, it's time now to think beyond the chemicals to seek sustainable and safe alternatives to cope with bacterial infections.

The viral predators, 'bacteriophages' can be the most suitable and potential alternative to cope with bacterial diseases.Phage therapy has been visited as one of seven approaches to "achieving a coordinated and nimble approach to addressing antibacterial resistance threats" in a 2014 status report from the National Institute of Allergy and Infectious Diseases (NIAID). That showed the importance of phage therapy as potential tool for fighting against the drug resistant bacteria. However, the success of phage therapy depends on our ability to overcome the limitations of using them as a therapeutic agent.

Bacteriophages

Bacteriophages are the most abundant organisms on the Earth. They are ubiquitous, obligate intracellular parasites and attack on the host cell, hijack the machinery and finally destroy it. Achaea and cyanobacteria are also attack by a group of viruses often called as cyanophages.Bacteriophages widely occur in, sewage, soil, water and marine water etc.

Structurally, most of bacteriophages consist of three parts i.e. head, tail and tail fiber. The head encloses nucleic acid which can be either DNA or RNA but not both. The tail is like a hollow tube through which nucleic acid passes in to the host cytosol during infection and tail fibers help bacteriophages to attach on the bacterial surface.

The size of most bacteriophages in general ranges from 22-200nm in length, while the largest bacteriophage known is T4 which is about 200nm long and 80-100nm wide.The most important feature of phages is their narrow host range i.e. they kill only specific bacterial strain and that makes them as potential antimicrobial agents.

This feature of bacteriophages is very advantageous because unlike broad-spectrum antibiotics, phage can kill specific pathogenic bacteria without he balance of beneficial bacterial microflora. However one drawback of this narrow bacteriophage host range isthat, bacteria may develop resistance against bacteriophage.

To solve this problem, phage "cocktail" i.e. a mixture of different bacteriophages are used that provides a wider antimicrobial range (6). Normally lytic bacteriophages infect and kill specific bacteria and are widely used in therapy because they act on short period of time. Furthermore, the mode of antimicrobial action of bacteriophages is very complex than mechanism of action of antibiotics.

Therefore in this chapter we are highlighting the use of bacteriophages as an alternative antimicrobial therapy and also other potential applications of bacteriophages.

Life cycle of bacteriophages

The bacteriophages display two types of life cycle i.e. lytic cycle and lysogenic cycle. In lytic cycle, bacteriophage attach on bacteria through various cell surface receptors such as lipopolysaccharids (LPS), teichoic acids and various structural proteins (OmpA, C and F) on bacterial cell wall and injects its nucleic acid into the cytosol.

Soon after, phage nucleic acid hijack the whole bacterial synthetic machinery that direct synthesis of phage specific mRNA, structural proteins and various other components. Later on, different phage components are assembled to form mature viral particles that come out from cell by lysis of the cell wall.

Approximately, a total of about 1000 viral particles may be released per cycle. In lysogenic cycle, phage nucleic acids get integrate in to the bacterial genome and replicate along with genome and passed on to the daughter cells. The integrated viral genome is called 'prophase' and this process is known as lysogeny. Under certain condition like high radiation, change in metabolism, stresses, phage genome gets excised and becomes a lytic phage.

Bacteriophages were discovered independently by a British microbiologist Frederick Twort in 1915 and Felix de Herelle (13, 14) however, the concept of bacteriophage therapy was introduced by Felix de Herelle in 1920.

Many countries like France, Georgia and United States and in Europe there are several phage therapy centers are working, and dealing with various human diseases. The extensive work on phage therapy was carried out between 1920 to 1930 in USA to treat infection caused by Streptococcus and Bacilli, "Staphylogel" and bacteriophage "gel labaled" preparation were manufactured by Eli Lilly and Company.

At the same time, antibiotics were discovered and widely used that causes rejection of bacteriophages as therapeutic agent in many countries include Europe and USA. Many papers have published between 1950 to 1980 that showed benefits of bacteriophage therapy in animal models.

Due to increase antibiotics resistance in bacteria, bacteriophage therapy was "rediscovered" with the work done by Smith and Huggins in 1980s. Now treatment of infection by phage was widely used in several countries namely Poland, United States, Europe (Georgia) and Russia.

Poland-The Hirszfeld Institute of Immunology and Experimental Therapy in Wroclaw was established in 1954 in which thousand patients were successfully treated with phages. For each patient phages were selected and prepared and treatment was done by specialized physician. The 75% to

100% cure rates for specific infection types were reported.

After the successful treatment of severe antibiotic resistance infections, the Institute itself opens a phage therapy center in 2005. United States-In US, phage therapy was started during 1920s and 1930s and treatment of chronic furonculsis was carried out by the Michigan Department of Health where phage administered subcutaneously.

Georgia- George Eliava established George Institute in Tbilisi in 1930s in which phage therapy was started in association of Felix d, Herelle. One pathogenic bacteria strain was received from the Soviet Union and phages were isolated from different sources, tested and administered against this bacterial strain.

Particularly the bacteriophage Sb-1 was found to be quite effective in eliminating MRSA infections. The Sb-1 bacteriophage was found to be effective against MRSA strains and in a case study involving a young cystic fibrosis patient infected with MRSA, treatment with the Sb-1 bacteriophage reduced MRSA levels below the limit of detection.

Russia- In addition to the above, Russia also play important role in the development of phage therapy. In Russia, diarrheal infection, gas gangrene and also infection of infants and child were successfully treated with phage therapy.

Bacteriophages were used in the form of tablets, creams, liquids and Russia is the first country where stable more effective tablet forms of bacteriophage was developed.

Why we need phage therapy?

The emergence of antibiotic –resistance bacteria has becomes a major problem for clinician over the last 2-3 decades. In United State, antibiotic resistance bacteria infect approximately 2 million people each year in which at least 23,000 people die annually. At present, most of the bacteria such as Acinetobacter baumannii, Staphylococcus aureus, Pseudomonas aeruginosa, Enterococus faecium, Klebsiella pneumonia have becomes multi-drug resistance and cause major healthcare crisis in ICUs.

The number of newly approved antibiotics have decreases in United State since 1980s and development of new antibiotics becomes unprofitable due to underlying economic condition and probably most of the newly developed antibiotic becomes ineffective soon after their introduction.

The development of severe new infectious disease caused by multidrug resistance bacteria that are not cure by antibiotics requires alternatives to classical antibiotics. Due to steadily declined discovery of new class of antibiotics, there is an urgent need to investigate new antimicrobial drugs. Therefore, bacteriophage may be used as therapeutic agent to treat infections caused by multi-drug resistance bacteria.

Advantages of Bacteriophage over Antibiotics

Bacteriophages are the potential unique therapeutic agents that have many advantages over classical antibiotics. Some most important advantages are given in the following table. Apart from those generalized advantages there are many specific advantages that the phage therapy has like 'Auto dosing'.

Phages during the bacterial-killing process are capable of increasing in number specifically where hosts are located, so phages are intelligent enough to put a desire dose to kill host bacteria i.e. we called it auto dosing. Low inherent toxicity, since phages consist mostly of nucleic acids and proteins, they are inherently nontoxic.

The relatively narrow host range exhibited by most phages limits the number of bacterial types with which selection for specific phage-resistance mechanisms can occur. Thus there is low pressure of resistance associated with phage therapy.

Because phages infect and kill using mechanisms that differ from those of anti-biotics, specific antibiotic resistance mechanisms do not translate into mechanisms of phage resistance

1 Bacteriophages are very specific means they targeted specific bacterial strains without affecting the normal beneficial bacterial micro flora of the body. Most of the antibiotics are broad spectrum .In addition to killing specific pathogenic bacteria; they also destroyed the normal beneficial micro- flora of the body. Thus they disturb microbial balance and may cause severe side effects.

2 When a bacterium becomes resistance to specific bacteriophage then it is very easy to find new bacteriophages against that bacterium.If a bacterium becomes resistance to an antibiotic ,it is very difficult to develop new antibiotic and this development process is very tedious and take many years

3 Many antibiotics cause allergies in several patients; in this case infections are successfully treated with bacteriophage therapy.Cure of infection will be very difficult if the patients are allergic to antibiotics.

4 Manufacture process of bacteriophage is very easy and cost effective. Manufacture process of antibiotics is costly, complex and time taken.

5 Bacteriphages have unique ability to multiply and increase their number at the site of infection thus treatment can be performed with very small dose. Antibiotics do not

accumulated at the site of infection; they are normally metabolized in the body and removed from the body through urine.

6 Multi-drug resistance (MDR) bacteria are easily treated with bacteriophages therapy. If the bacteria become multi-drug resistance, treatment with antibiotics will be very difficult.

7 Bacteriophages are nontoxic to human thus; there are no severe side effects. Use of antibiotic cause severe side effects includes allergic reaction, intestinal disorders and several secondary infections.

6. Bacteriophages as antimicrobial Bacteriophage therapy is widely used to treat severe infections caused by multi-drug resistance pathogenic bacteria in human ,animals and plants and it is now also employ to enhance the shelf –life of meats, vegetables, fruits and stored plant parts.

Bacteriophage isolation, purification and preparations of commercial phage

Bacteriophages can be easily isolated from their natural sources such as water, soil, sewage, fermented product and unprocessed vegetables following standard protocol. This is the first step of any phage therapy protocol. After isolation, purification was performed by using filtration, ultracentrifugation, polyethylene glycol method and various forms of chromatography.

The above methods normally removed ruptured bacterial ghost cells, uninfected cells and other components of bacteria. Several phage preparations were developed by Eli Lilly Company against Syaphylococci, Streptococci, E. coli and for various other infectious pathogenic bacteria for the human use. Important example of commercially obtainable bacteriophage preparations includes

Ento-lysate, Staphylo-lysate, Neiso-lysate and Colo-lysate. Diabetic wounds, chronic infections, upper respiratory tract infection, abscesses and various otherinfections are successfully treated by using these phage preparations (20). D'Herelle's commercial laboratory in Paris produced at least five phage preparations against various bacterial infections.

The preparations were called as Bactécoli-phage, Bacté-rhino-phage, Bacté-intesti-phage, Bacté-pyo-phage, and Bacté-staphy-phage, and they were marketed by the French company L'Oréal later on. In the 1940s, the Eli Lilly Company (Indianapolis, Ind.) in United States, produced seven phage products for human use, targeted against Staphylococci, Streptococci, Escherichia coli, and other bacterial pathogens.

Mainly these preparations contains phage-lysed, sterile cultures of the host bacteria (e.g., Cololysate, Ento-lysate, Neiso-lysate, and Staphylo-lysate) or the same preparations in a water-soluble jelly base (e.g., Colojel, Ento-jel, and Staphylo-jel). They were used to treat various infections, including abscesses, suppurating wounds,vaginitis, acute and chronic infections of the upper respiratory tract, and mastoid infections.

Mode of delivery of bacteriophages

The success of bacteriophage-derived therapeutics and biosensors will ultimately rely on suitably robust, reproducible, delivery technologies. Delivery of suitably-engineered phage has permitted isolation of allergens inducing IgE production using high throughput screening technologies.

Phages can also be engineered to bear target-specific peptides or proteins for biorecognition, and thus may have application in development of novel chemical and biological sensors that may provide quantitative or semi-quantitative data through exploitation of a chemical or biological recognition element.

The potential routes of administration of phages include topical, oral, rectal, and parenteral; topical administration to chronic wound infections is the most frequently reported route. In such infections, phage cocktails—combinations of avariety of phages—have been used.

One product used at the Eliava Institute is PhageBioDerm, a biodegradable polymer wound dressing impregnated with ciprofloxacin, benzocaine, chymotrypsin, bicarbonate, and 6 lytic phages (Pyophage) with activity against Pseudomonas aeruginosa, Staphylococcus aureus, Escherichia coli, Streptococcus species, and Proteus species.

Other potential means of topical administration include sprays, aerosols, lozenges, mouthwash, suppositories, bandages, eye drops, and tampons. Intrapleural administration and bladder irrigation are also feasible.

Oral administration of phage

Gastrointestinal infection and systemic infections are successfully treated with oral delivery of phage. The main difficulty with phage delivery through this route is that phage can be inactivated in the highly acidic condition of the stomach. To avoid such problem, polymer microencapsulated phages are used that protect phage from inactivation by acid and also enhance efficacy of phages. Other way of neutralizing acidity of stomach is use of sodium bicarbonate or sodium bicarbonate mineral water before administration of phages.

Local administration of phage

This is the most successful route of phage administration where phage suspensions directly apply on the infected area.In addition to above routes, phage can also be administered to human by intravenously (IV), intaperitonial (IP), intramuscular (IM), and subcutaneous (SC) methods.

Pharmacology and pharmacokinetics of phage therapy

The effect of drug's on the body as well as the body's impact on drugs is known as pharmacology. Pharmacokinetics is explanation of a drug's potential to arrive in the near of specific target cells or tissues which are enough to achieve primary pharmacodynamic effect.

This explanation is to differentiate in to distribution, absorption, metabolism as well as elimination of drugs. In case of bacteriophage, metabolism represents "inactivation" of phage because host immune system interacts and inactivates the phage or "activation" due to phage replication inside the host body.

For success of a phage therapy, generation of adequate number of phages is necessary in the immediate vicinity of specific target bacteria that cause pathogen eradication from the body at some adequate rate. Bacteriophage will increase their sufficient number through in situ replication in host body and so- called active treatment.

Thus the main goal pharmacologically is to gain sufficient densities of phages in the vicinity of target bacteria that lead to bacterial eradication.

Phage therapy in human

In human, several infectious diseases such as septicemia, wound infections, skin infection, osteomyelitis, urinary tract infections and middle ear infections were successfully treated with phage therapy. In many countries like US, phages were widely used for human and animal vaccine preparation. In phage therapy, phages were used in the form of liquid suspension, tablets, creams rinses, aerosols.

Bacteriophage safety

The description of toxicity of drugs and their impact on non-target tissues comes under the category of secondary pharmacodynamics. Many evidences clearly showed that bacteriophages interact with non-target cells and tissues of human. Several phages are taken up by gastrointestinal tract in to the blood stream and reticulo-endothelial system is also appears to interact with phages. However, interaction of phages with non-target tissues has no major side effect recorded so far.

The immunology of phages is not yet known extensively. When the phages delivered by intravenous route, they are quickly removed from circulatory system and predominantly stored in liver and spleen. Many evidences suggested that, the head proteins of bacteriophages interact with certain receptors found on the immune cells which result in cytokines production and humoral immune response while it is unclear that, phage stimulate cell-mediated immune response.

One of the most serious problems that have been displayed by phage therapy safety is that some phages (temperate phage) have unique ability to incorporate their genome and modify host bacteria that make them more potential pathogenic thus it is important to avoid temperate phage for therapy (27).

The U.S. Food and Drug Administration (FDA) did not have guidelines for reviewing bacteriophage preparations until recently, and those guidelines needs yet to finalize. Earlier FDA-approved clinical uses in the

1970s, 1980s, and 1990s involved phage phi x174, which was administered intravenously for nontherapeutic purposes to patients with Down syndrome, Wiskott-Aldrich syndrome, HIV infections, and other immunodeficiencies. FDA also conducted a safety review of bacteriophages in 1973 after phages were found in several vaccines.

Agency officials concluded that the vaccines were safe and allowed their continued use. That first U.S. trial also put lot of concern about developing phage therapies in humans that FDA officials might insist on single phage preparations instead of cocktails. The long-term efficacy of single-phage preparations is questionable, and early commercial failures could hinder development of phage therapy in the United States

Most phage therapy trials in the former Soviet Union and Eastern Europe have involved multivalent phage cocktails, according to published reports (Challenges in Developing Phage Therapies).

Improvement of phage therapy through modern techniques

Therapeutic and prophylactic application of bacteriophages are encouraging over conventional medicine, there is an obvious need to develop phage therapy in wide range of applications. Though the first reported discovery of antibacterial-like activity linked to bacteriophages was made in 1896, where Ernest Hanbury Hankin stated that the waters of the Ganga and Jamuna rivers might have restricted outbreaks of cholera.

Since then due to lack of information regarding basic phage biology and early antibacterial drugs together restricted the development of phage therapy. In recent years due to increased threat of bacterial resistance to drugs and lack of new antibacterial drug development, opened new opportunities to develop phase therapy. Moreover with increased information regarding

phage biology and improvements in molecular biology researchers have now progressed to the point where sufficient knowledge acquired to improve phase therapy as next-generation application.

Development of genetically engineered bacteriophages

Genetic engineering helps to improve the phase therapy to overcome many obstacles involved in using wild type phases. While treating gram-negative bacteria cell wall liberates endotoxin which is harmful and cause bacterimia, septicemia etc.

To overcome this difficulty, several bacteriophages have now been developed through genetic engineering that are non-replicating and non-lytic. These genetic engineered bacteriophage, encode specific proteins that are deleterious to bacteria with release of only small amount of endotoxin. Helicobacter pylori and Pseudomonas aeruginosa infection are successfully treated with these genetically engineered and non-replicating bacteriophags.

Engineered bacteriophage can enhance the killing of antibiotic-resistant bacteria, persister cells, and biofilm cells,reduce the number of antibiotic-resistant bacteria that arise from an antibiotic-treated population, and act as a strong adjuvant for other bactericidal antibiotics.. Host range of a T7 phage incresed by expression of an endosial-idase which degrades the K1 capsule present in some E. coli strains, thereby allowing the modified T7 to surpass this barrier, enhancing phage adsorption to efficiently infect K1 E. coli.

Cock tail of phages that are genetically modified would be more helpful in addressing a wide variety of bacterial infections that are otherwise resistant to the latest generations of antibiotics. SOS gene networks of E. coli was inactivated by the use of genetically engineered bacteriophages, enhance the capability of antibiotics such as ß-lactams, quinolones, aminoglycosides to works on bacteria quickly and more effectively. Likewise many researchers are using genetic engineering approach to advance the phase therapy

Genetic engineered bacteriophage as adjuvant

There are many genes in bacterial genome whose products are harmful to human on which antibiotics cannot target directly. Therefore, genetic engineered bacteriophages were developed that have ability to overexpress proteins to target the bacterial gene networks on which the antibiotics cannot works and increases destruction of bacteria by antibiotics.

With recent advances of DNA synthesis, synthetic phages were developed and well-suited for incorporating targets, identified via systems biology, in a modular fashion to create effective antibiotic adjuvants. These everimproving technologies will enable large-scale modifications of phage libraries to produce antibiotic-adjuvant phage that target different gene networks and that can be applied with different antibiotic drugs against a wide range of bacteria.

Combination therapy which couples antibiotics with engineered antibiotic adjuvant phage is a promising antimicrobial strategy for the future.

Use of phage lytic enzymes

Many bacteriophages posses' lytic enzymes such as holins and lysins that have ability to battle against host to survive. They have yet to be exploited. Now new techniques are employed in which bacteriophages are used in combination with phage lytic enzymes that enhance the killing capacity of bacteriophages.

All of these enzymes are highly evolved molecules designed for a specific purpose, to quickly destroy the bacterial cell wall, and as such, nanogram quantities of enzyme are sufficient to sterilize a 107 bacterial suspension in seconds. Because of the serious problems of resistant bacteria in hospitals, day care centers, and nursing homes, particularly Staphylococci and Pneumococcal, such enzymes may be of immediate benefit in these environments.

Thus, we may add phage enzymes to our armamentarium against pathogenic bacteria.

Other potential applications of bacteriophages

In addition to phage therapy, bacteriophages are also being employed for phage display, phage typing, vehicles for vaccine delivery, targeted gene delivery, bio-control, eradication of biofilm and food industry.

Phage display

Phage display was likely the first phage application as a tool of modern biotechnology (53). The term phage display was first introduced in 1985. Phage display is a unique molecular technique in which exogenous proteins are expressed on the surface of a bacteriophage.

In phage display technique, desired gene that encodes the protein is fused with phage coat-protein gene and is displayed on the surface of bacteriophage. Through phage display technique, novel phages are developed, these phages have a variety of applications. Escherichia coli filamentous phage M13 is most extensively used in phage display but other phages such as lambda phage of E.coli and T7 Phage have also been widely used.

By the use of phage display, a specific protein or antibody can be purifying because specific phages are very easy and cost effective to purify. The various applications of phage display include mapping of epitopes, in vaccine design, in study of protein-protein interaction, in determination of specificity of enzymes and inhibitors, in screening for anti-cancer peptide and proteins and in screening for receptors.

Phage typing

Bacteriophages are very specific to their host means a bacteriophage especially infect and destroy only one or a few type of bacteria. This specificity of phages for bacterial cells are widely used for the detection of pathogenic bacteria and for bacterial strain typing, a technique known as phage typing.

In Phage typing the lawn of unknown bacterial strains, is provided with various different phages, when the phages infect and lysed specific bacterial strains clear zones (plaques) appear on the lawn, in this way specific bacterial strains can be easily detected. In addition to phage typing,

other techniques are also widely used for the detection of pathogenic bacteria such as use of green fluorescent proteins and use of phages that deliver reporter genes specifically.

Phages as vehicles for vaccine delivery

Bacteriophages have been widely used as vehicles for the delivery of vaccines (59). They are employed in the two ways, one in which phages can be used directly, bearing vaccine antigens display on their surfaces and other in DNA vaccine, the gene or sequences that synthesized vaccine antigen firstly incorporated in to the phage genome then phage would act as vehicles for the delivery of DNA vaccine.

Targeted gene delivery through phages

Bacteriophages have also been widely used as specific gene delivery vectors. The phages employ in this purpose is similar to that for using phages for DNA vaccine delivery. The foreign proteins expressed on the surface of bacteriophage that enable them targeting specific cell types and after injection, phage coat protein save DNA from degradation, which is a prerequisite for successful gene therapy.

Phages as bio-control agents

Bacteriophages are widely used as bio-control of plant pathogens. Many plant pathogens such as Xanthomonas pruni that infect cabbage, peppers, and peaches, Ralstonia solanacearum cause disease in Tobacco, Xanthomonas comprestris cause spots on tomatoes, Pseudomonas talaasi cause blotch of mushrooms have been successfully control by bacteriophages.

Eradication of biofilm by phages

Biofilms are aggregation of microorganisms, growing either on living or non-living surfaces and secrete huge amount of extracellular polymers (EPS) that surround them. Environmental conditions stimulate most of the bacteria to form biofilms and biofilms formation is an important strategy of bacterial survival. Biofilms formation cause severe disease in human and is resistance to antibiotics and host immune systems.

Because biofilms are resistance to antimicrobial drugs, therefore alternative therapy must be needed to control biofilm-associated diseases. Evidences suggest that, bacteriophages efficiently eradicate biofims.

Phages in food industry

Many pathogenic bacteria have contaminated the foods which result in foodborn disease. At present, leading cause of death due to the foodborn pathogens are Listeria and Salmonella and followed by E.coli and Campylobacter jejunii. Bacteriophages give effective and safe means to eradicate the food born pathogenic bacteria that contaminate the foods.

Major obstacles of phage therapy

Although it seems everything in favor of using lytic phages as therapeutics but they are not commonly used to the extent of expectations and sometimes their efficacy is a matter of controversy. One of the most significant factors associated with the efficacy of phage therapy is the paucity of a appropriate placebo-controlled studies. Here is some major obstacle in the application of phage therapy.

1. Heterogeneity and ecology of both phages and bacteria

2. Selection of highly virulent phages against targeted host bacteria

3. Monophage preparations against different bacteria

4. Selective phage cocktail appropriately characterize or titre phage preparations

5. Genetically engineered phages

6. Lateral gene transfer of virulence factors and antibiotic resistance

7. Restriction modification degradation of phage DNA upon infection

8. Resistance mutations in bacterial genes for adsorption, lysogeny and lysogenic conversion

9. Phage-host interactions

10. Phage preparation and characterization i.e. to determine the virulence to the target

11. Neutralize gastric pH prior to oral administration

12. Immunogenicity antibodies developed against phage

13. Endotoxins in phage preparation

14. Phage reprogramming

Rapid clearance of bacteriophages

The quick removal of bacteriophages by liver, spleen and other different filtering organs of reticuloendothelial system lowers the densities of phages to a level, this lower concentration of phages is not sufficient to combat against infections.

Generation of antibodies against bacteriophages

When the phages administered intravenously, humoral immune system activated which result in production of antibodies. These phage specific antibodies rapidly inactivate the phages. This is the major obstacles for phage therapy. However, antibodies are not produced, if local and oral route of administration used. The issue of bacteriophage interactions with the mammalian immune system and its components is still not precisely defined.

Evidence increasingly suggests that phages influence mammalian immune responses, including the attenuation of specific and nonspecific immune reactions, and maintenance of local immune tolerance to gut microorganism-derived antigens.

Although innate immunity cannot be entirely separated from its adaptive counterpart, for the purpose of clarity, we will also discuss antiphage immunity according to the mechanism(s) of neutralization and clearance.

Intracellular pathogens

Many pathogens such as Mycobacterium tuberculosis, Salmonella Typhimurium, Rickettsia, and Chlamydia etc. are intracellular means they multiply inside the host cells and make pathogens inaccessible by phages. Thus the infections caused by these intracellular bacteria cannot be treated by bacteriophages. Therefore use of bacteriophage is limited in case of intracellular pathogens.

Narrow host range of phage

The bacteriophage has narrow host range. When patients are infected with multiple bacteria, in this situation bacteriophage therapy will not effective.

Development of resistance

Like human immune system bacteria also have innate immune system (e.g. Restriction –modification (R-M) system and acquired immune system (e.g. CRISPR-Cas system) that cleave and destroy phage DNA entering in to cells. Thus bacteria developed resistance against bacteriophages, which result in failure of phage therapy.

In addition to above, phage preparations contain bacterial derbies and endotoxins, failure to establish scientific proof of efficacy and development of lysogeny limits the use of phage therapy.

Future directions

There is increasing interest in 'Phage therapy' as possible new drug with hope to cope with multi drug resistance bacterial infections. Despite approval of some phage formulation by agencies like FDA, US-FSIS and GRAS in various applications in the field of food and biomedical sectors, there still a lot of concerns associated for their commercial acceptance.

If not carrying a variance factor most of phages are supposed to be safe for human beings, but increasing efforts to make recombinant viral particles raises several biosafety concerns over possibility of bringing new genetic traits in bacterial populations. So, new methods must be developed to reprogram the phages without any genetic modifications to possess auxiliary mechanisms for phage adherence/binding and uptake that are critical for plaque formation.

Another core area that need more focus in phage therapy is to allow a better selection of lytic phages for reprogramming them. This should be capable of converting naturally occurring wild phages into smart phages with a broader range of host specificity that can overcome a bacterial defense mechanisms. These findings encourage new optimism and a re-evaluation of the potential for phage therapy.

War against Antibiotic Resistant Bacteria

Bacteriophages or phages are bacterial viruses that invade bacterial cells and, in the case of lytic phages, disrupt bacterial metabolism and cause the bacterium to lyse.Recent examples of the use of bacteriophages in controlling bacterial infections are presented, some of which show therapeutic promise.

The therapeutic use of bacteriophages, possibly in combination with antibiotics, may be a valuable approach. However, it is also quite clear that the safe and controlled use of phage therapy will require detailed information on the properties and behavior of specific phage–bacterium systems, both in vitro and especially in vivo.

In vivo susceptibility of bacterial pathogens to bacteriophages is still largely poorly understood and future research on more phage–bacterium systems has to be undertaken to define the requirements for successful phage treatments.

The emergence of pathogenic bacteria resistant to most, if not all, currently available antimicrobial agents has become a critical problem in modern medicine, particularly because of the concomitant increase in immunosuppressed patients.

The concern that humankind is reentering the "preantibiotics" era has become very real, and the development of alternative ant infection modalities has become one of the highest priorities of modern medicine and biotechnology.

Viruses that attack bacteria were observed by Twort and d'Herelle in 1915 and 1917. They observed that broth cultures of certain intestinal bacteria could be dissolved by addition of a bacteria-free filtrate obtained from sewage. The lysis of the bacterial cells was said to be brought about by a virus which meant a "filterable poison"

Probably every known bacterium is subject to infection by one or more viruses or "bacteriophages" as they are known ("phage" for short, from Gr. "phagein" meaning "to eat" or "to nibble"). Most research has been done on the phages that attack E. coli, especially the T-phages and phage lambda. Like most viruses, bacteriophages typically carry only the genetic information needed for replication of their nucleic acid and synthesis of their protein coats. When phages infect their host cell, the order of business is to replicate their nucleic acid and to produce the protective protein coat. But they cannot do this alone. They require precursors, energy generation and ribosomes supplied by their bacterial host cell.

Bacterial cells can undergo one of two types of infections by viruses termed lytic infections and lysogenic (temperate) infections. In E. coli, lytic infections are caused by a group seven phages known as the T-phages, while lysogenic infections are caused by the phage lambda.

Lytic Infections

The T-phages, T1 through T7, are referred to as lytic phages because they always bring about the lysis and death of their host cell, the bacterium E. coli. T-phages contain double-stranded DNA as their genetic material. In addition to their protein coat or capsid (also referred to as the "head"), T-phages also possess a tail and some related structures.

Before viral infection, the cell is involved in replication of its own DNA and transcription and translation of its own genetic information to carry out biosynthesis, growth and cell division. After infection, the viral DNA takes over the machinery of the host cell and uses it to produce the nucleic acids and proteins needed for production of new virus particles.

Viral DNA replaces the host cell DNA as a template for both replication (to produce more viral DNA) and transcription (to produce viral mRNA). Viral mRNAs are then translated, using host cell ribosomes, tRNAs and amino acids, into viral proteins such as the coat or tail proteins. The process of DNA replication, synthesis of proteins, and viral assembly is a carefully coordinated and timed event.

Before viral infection, the cell is involved in replication of its own DNA and transcription and translation of its own genetic information to carry out biosynthesis, growth and cell division. After infection, the viral DNA takes over the machinery of the host cell and uses it to produce the nucleic acids and proteins needed for production of new virus particles. Viral DNA replaces the host cell DNA as a template for both replication (to produce more viral DNA) and transcription (to produce viral mRNA). Viral mRNAs are then translated, using host cell ribosomes, tRNAs and amino acids, into viral proteins such as the coat or tail proteins. The process of DNA replication, synthesis of proteins, and viral assembly is a carefully coordinated and timed event.

Phage Therapy

Phage therapy is the therapeutic use of lytic bacteriophages to treat pathogenic bacterial infections. Phage therapy is an alternative to antibiotics being developed for clinical use by research groups in Eastern Europe and the U.S. After having been extensively used and developed mainly in former Soviet Union countries for about 90 years, phage therapies for a variety of bacterial and poly microbial infections are now becoming available on an experimental basis in other countries, including the U.S. The principles of phage therapy have potential applications not only in human medicine, but also in dentistry, veterinary science, food science and agriculture.

An important benefit of phage therapy is derived from the observation that bacteriophages are much more specific than most antibiotics that are in clinical use. Theoretically, phage therapy is harmless to the eukaryotic host undergoing therapy, and it should not affect the beneficial normal flora of the host. Phage therapy also has few, if any, side effects, as opposed to drugs, and does not stress the liver. Since phages are self-replicating in their target bacterial cell, a single, small dose is theoretically efficacious.

On the other hand, this specificity may also be disadvantageous because a specific phage will only kill a bacterium if it is a match to the specific subspecies. Thus, phage mixtures may be applied to improve the chances of success, or clinical samples can be taken and an appropriate phage identified and grown.Phages are currently being used therapeutically to treat bacterial infections that do not respond to conventional antibiotics, particularly in the country of Georgia. They are reported to be especially successful where bacteria have constructed a biofilm composed of a polysaccharide matrix that antibiotics cannot penetrate.

Bacterial Host Specificity

The bacterial host range of phage is generally narrower than that found in the antibiotics that have been selected for clinical applications. Most phage are specific for one species of bacteria and many are only able to lyse specific strains within a species.

This limited host range can be advantageous, in principle, as phage therapy results in less harm to the normal body flora and ecology than commonly used antibiotics, which often disrupt the normal gastrointestinal flora and result in opportunistic secondary infections by organisms such as Clostridium difficile.

The potential clinical disadvantages associated with the narrow host range of most phage strains is addressed through the development of a large collection of well-characterized phage for a broad range of pathogens, and methods to rapidly determine which of the phage strains in the collection will be effective for any given infection.

Advantages Over Antibiotics

Phage therapy can be very effective in certain conditions and has some unique advantages over antibiotics. Bacteria also develop resistance to phages, but it is incomparably easier to develop new phage than new antibiotic. A few weeks versus years are needed to obtain new phage for new strain of resistant bacteria. As bacteria evolve resistance, the relevant phages naturally evolve alongside. When super bacterium appears, the super phage already attacks it.

We just need to derive it from the same environment. Phages have special advantage for localized use, because they penetrate deeper as long as the infection is present, rather than decrease rapidly in concentration below the surface like antibiotics.

The phages stop reproducing once as the specific bacteria they target are destroyed. Phages do not develop secondary resistance, which is quite often in antibiotics. With the increasing incidence of antibiotic resistant bacteria and a deficit in the development of new classes of antibiotics to counteract them, there is a need to apply phages in a range of infections.

Advantages of bacteriophage Therapy

1. For every type of bacteria known in nature, there is at least one complementary bacteriophage that specifically infects a single bacterial species. So bacteriophage therapy is possible in all bacterial infections.

2. If a suitable bacteriophage is introduced onto an infected wound, it will continue to increase in numbers as long as there are bacteria to infect and destroy. However, as soon as all the bacteria have been destroyed, the action of the phage will cease and the dormant phage particles will disperse harmlessly.

3. Because phages are so specific to the bacteria they infect, they will not harm other beneficial bacteria present in the intestine and other parts of the body and will not affect the microbial ecosystem in the body.

There is no chance ofsuper infection with other bacteria. The bacterial imbalance caused by treatment with many antibiotics can lead to serious secondary infections involving relatively resistant bacteria, often extending hospitalization time, expense and mortality. This will not occur with specific bacteriophage therapy.

4. Some people are allergic to antibiotics so phage therapy could be a useful alternative for these patients. No patienthas ever been known to suffer an allergic reaction to bacteriophages. That may be because phages are omnipresent living organisms on earth, found in soil, water, plants and humans.

5. Phage therapies can be administered to patients in different ways which include pills, injections, enemas, nasal sprays, ointments, etc.

6. Each phage infects a specific bacteria or range of bacteria. A person in hospital, where bacterial infections abound, can be treated with a range of phages targeted at several types of bacteria. They can be given a cocktail of phage types to attack one type of bacteria or they can be given a combination of phage and antibiotic treatment.

7. Phages are considered safe for therapeutic use. No major side effects have been described so far. Only a very few side effects have been reported in the patients undergoing phage therapy. This might be related to extensive liberation of endotoxins from dead bacteria as the phages were destroying the bacteria most effectively. This type of reaction can also happen when antibiotics are used.

11. Since selection of active phages is a natural process, evolutionary arguments support the idea that active phage can be selected against every resistant bacterium, by an ever ongoing process of natural selection.

12. Production is simple and relatively inexpensive. So the treatment costs of bacterial infections will be reduced. This facilitates their potential applications to underserved populations.

Problems associated with bacteriophage therapy

1. Because of the high specificity of phages, the disease-causing bacterium has to be identified before the administration of phage therapy. One phage kills only aspecific subgroup of bacteria. One species of bacteria may contain many subgroups. But one antibiotic may kill many different species and subgroups of bacteria simultaneously. So a physician would need to make a specific diagnosis before prescribing a phage treatment.

2. Absences of bacteriophage action efficacy in certain cases were reported. It may be due to insufficient diagnostics and incorrect choice of the method for implementation of a specific phage.

3. The gastric acidity should be neutralized prior to oral phage administration.

4. Bacteriophage with a lytic lifecycle within a well-defined in vitro environment does not ensure that the bacteriophage will always remain lytic under normal physiological conditions found in a body. It may change to adapt lysogenic cycle in some circumstances.

5. Bacteriophages are viruses and, in general, viruses tend to swap genes with each other and other organisms with which they come into contact. So there is a chance of spread of antibiotic resistance in bacteria.

6. Many doctors are scared to give live bacteriophage to the patients.

Conclusion

Bacteriophages are a possible alternative tool for the treatment of bacterial infections, including those caused by MDR pathogens. Indeed, phage therapy displays several advantages and few adverse events are reported but underreporting cannot be ruled out. However, further well-conducted studies are required to define the role and safety of phage therapy in daily clinical practice to treat patients with various infections.

Moreover, direct use of phage encoded proteins such as endolysins, exopolysaccharidases and holins have proved their ability as a promising alternative to antibacterial products. This topic is, however, beyond the scope of this review.

Phages, as antibacterial agents, have a number of properties that make them compelling alternatives to chemical antibiotics while most or perhaps all concerns associated with phage therapy should be manageable through a combination of proper phage selection, effective formulation, and greater clinician understanding of and familiarity with product application.

Suitable phages, for example, were selected by characterizing their range of antibacterial virulence (narrow or broad), phage stability was confirmed at various temperatures, phage cocktails were developed to presumptively treat acute infections, and new phages were easily isolated against bacterial strains obtained from chronic infections.

In an era where antibiotic-resistant bacterial infections are on the rise, phages provide numerous advantages, along with relatively few disadvantages. In light of science now having a much greater understanding of phage biology along with higher standards for medical investigation than were the case during phage therapy's early, formative years,phage therapy merits a second chance within Western medicine to show its true potential.

The use of bacteriophages to control bacterial infections shows therapeutic promise. The worldwide increase of pathogenic bacteria resistant to antibiotics makes it an imperative to exploit alternative strategies to combat this threat. The therapeutic use of bacteriophages –perhaps in combination with antibiotics – may turn out to a valuable approach. However, it is also quite clear that the safe and controlled use of phage therapy will require detailed information on the properties and behavior of the specific phage–bacterium system, both in vitro and especially in vivo. The in vivo susceptibility of bacterial pathogens to bacteriophages is still largely poorly understood.